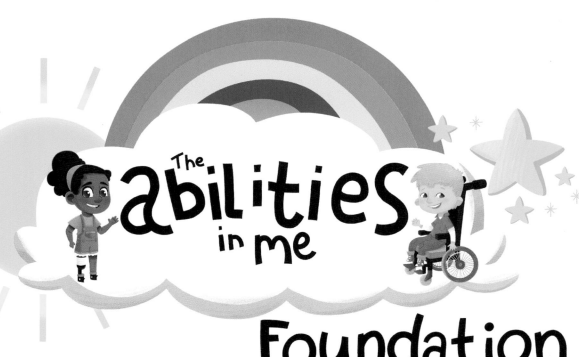

Foundation

www.theabilitiesinme.com

This book is dedicated to Ethan Sharma,
age 9 with Duchenne muscular dystrophy

Published in association with Bear With Us Productions

© 2021 Gemma Keir
The Abilities In Me - Superstar Siblings

www.theabilitiesinme.com

ISBN: 9798767770656

Edited by Emma Lusty and Claire Bunyan
Design by Luisa Moschetti
Illustrated by Novel Varius

www.justbearwithus.com

The abilities in me

Duchenne Muscular Dystrophy

Written by Gemma Keir

Illustrated by Novel Varius

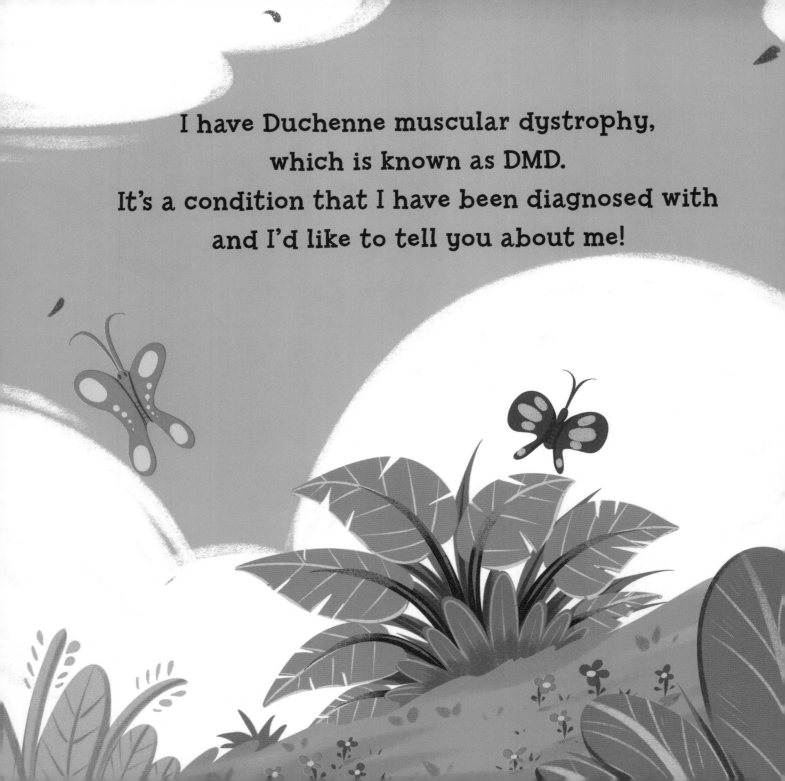

I have Duchenne muscular dystrophy,
which is known as DMD.
It's a condition that I have been diagnosed with
and I'd like to tell you about me!

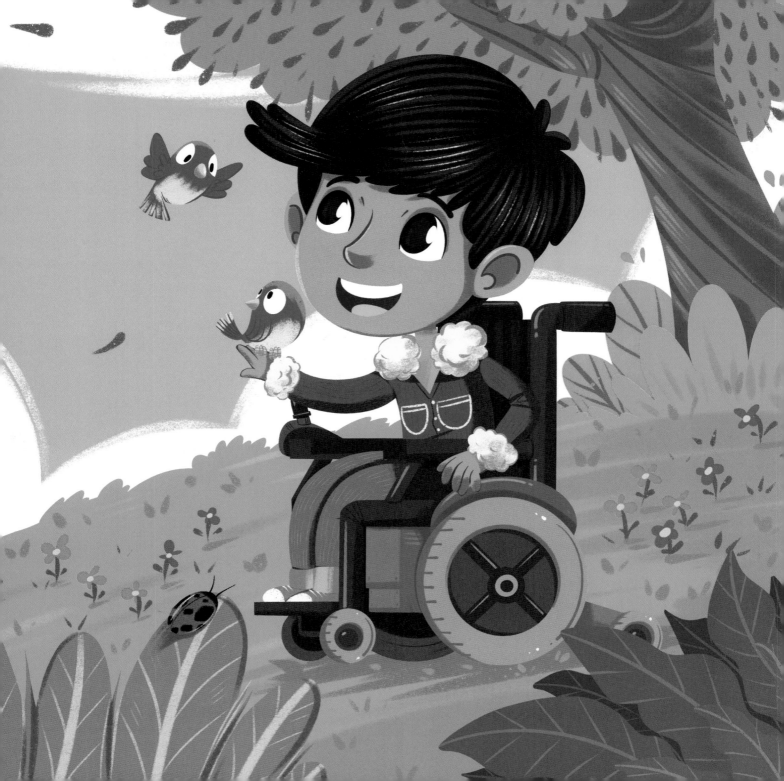

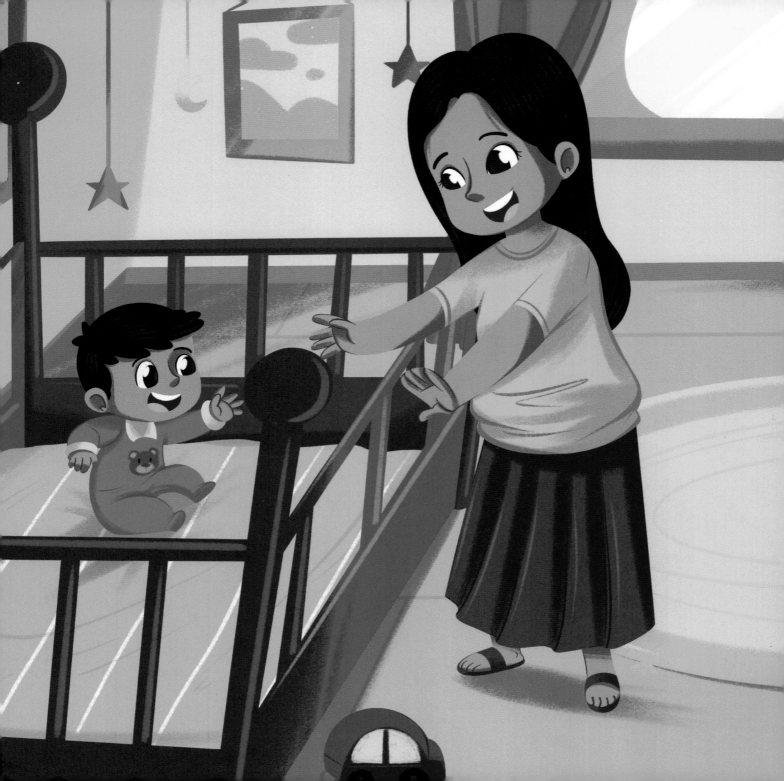

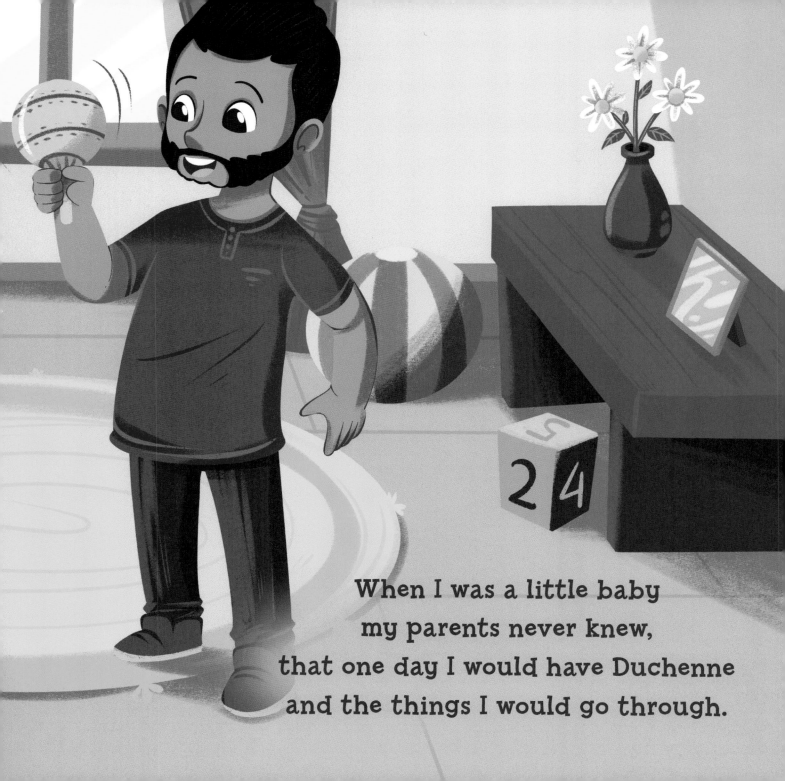

When I was a little baby
my parents never knew,
that one day I would have Duchenne
and the things I would go through.

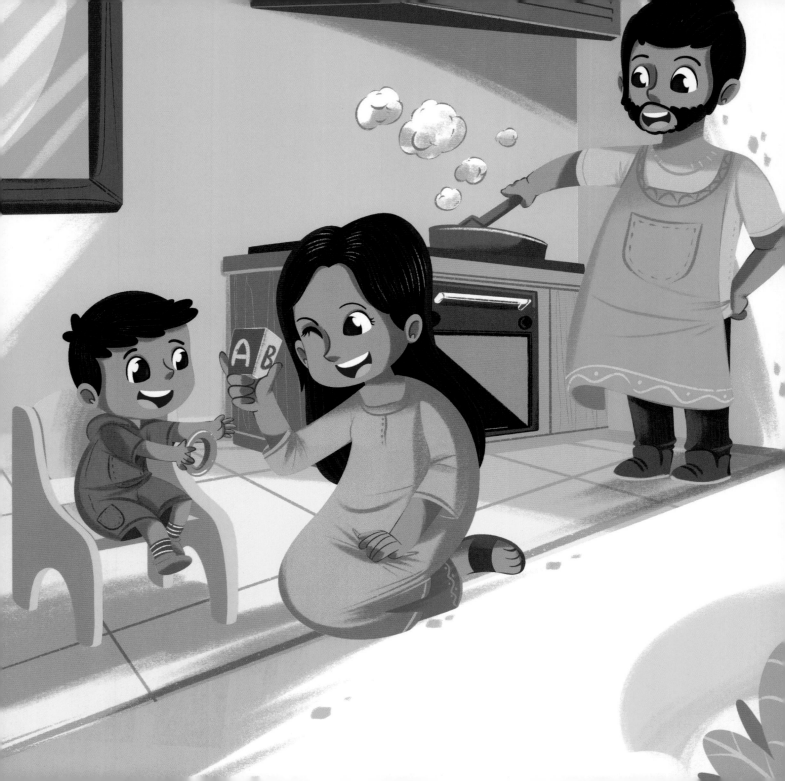

As I grew into a toddler,
I learned to grow and talk.
I loved to play with all my toys
and go on a nice family walk.

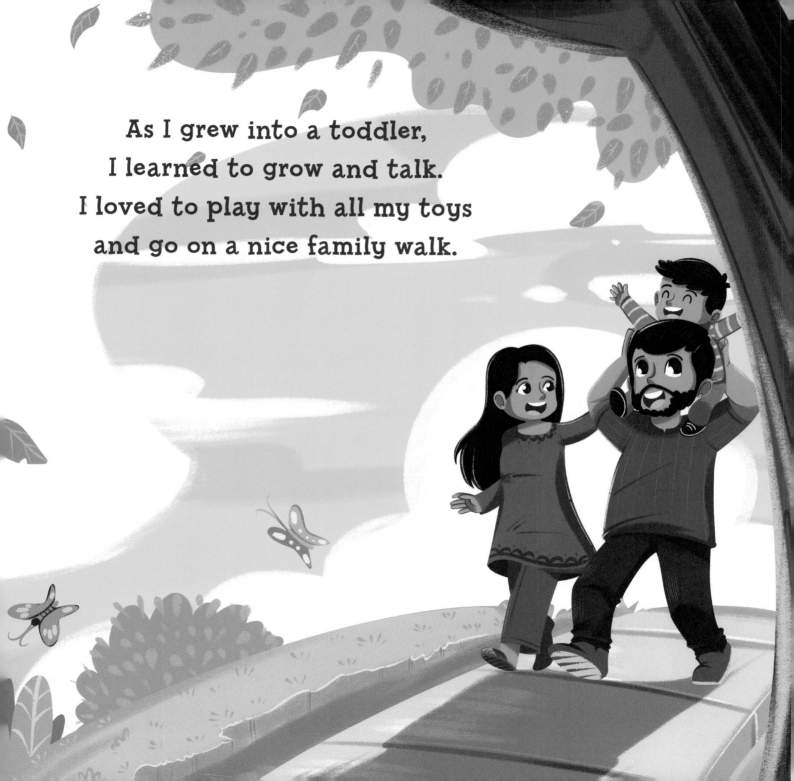

But then something started to happen,
I was feeling really tired and sore.

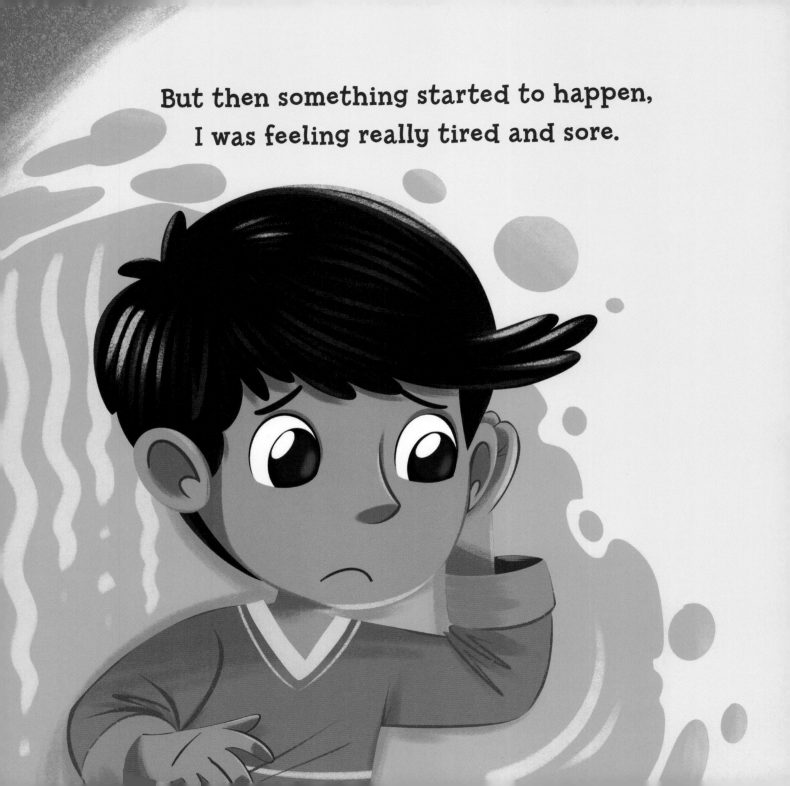

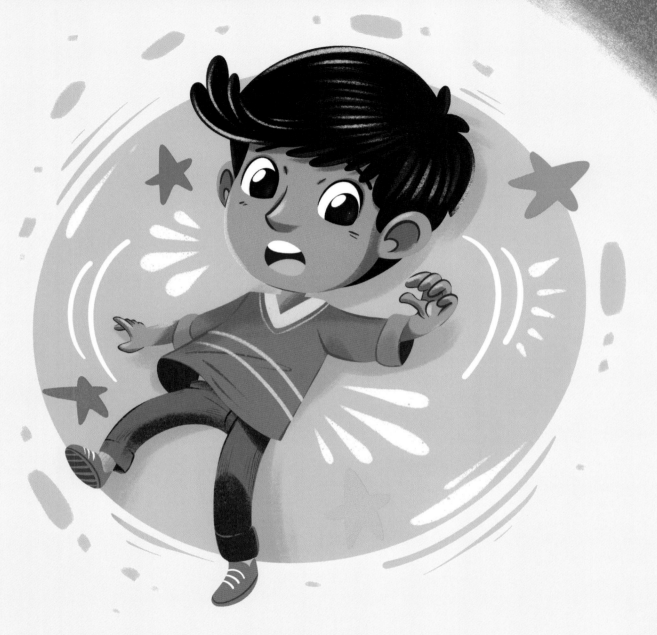

At times I would feel wobbly,
I would fall down to the floor.

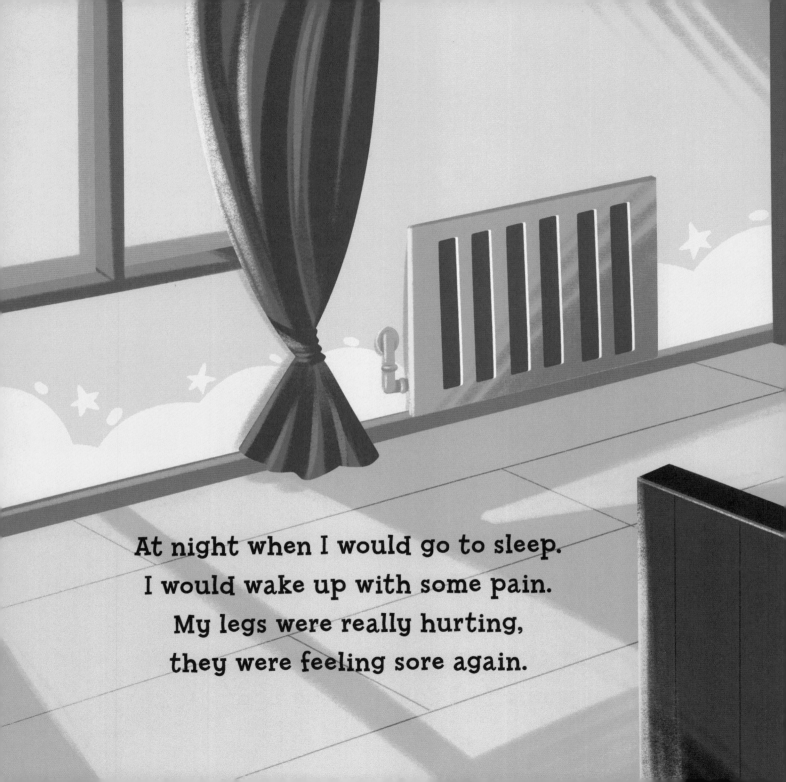

At night when I would go to sleep.
I would wake up with some pain.
My legs were really hurting,
they were feeling sore again.

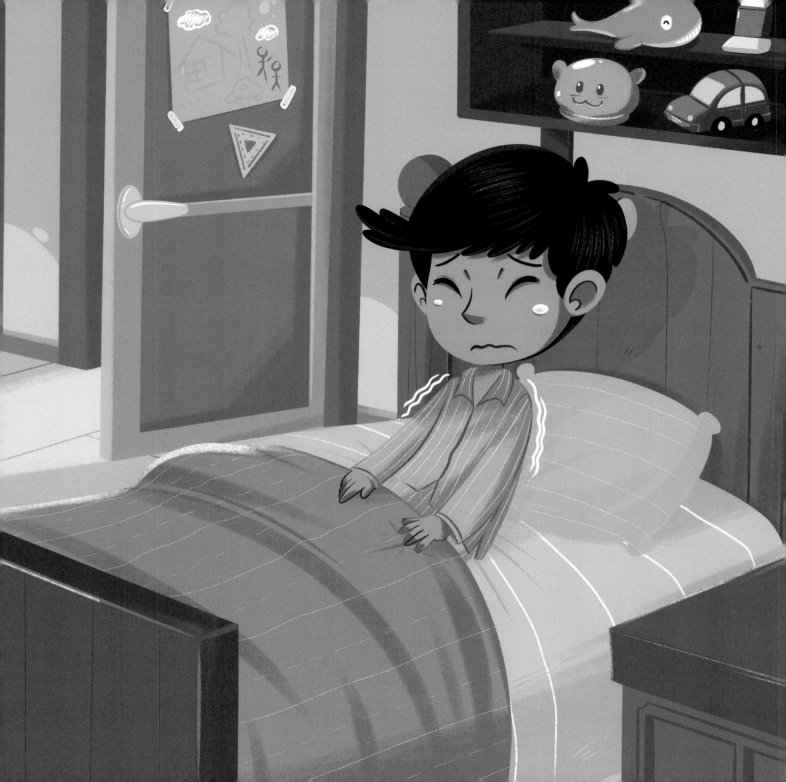

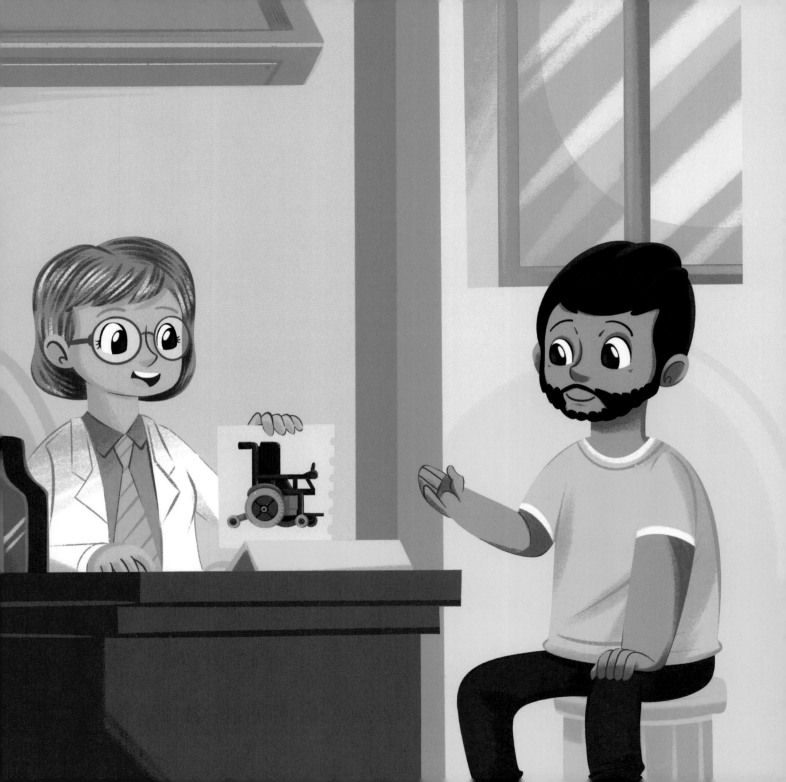

The doctor said I have DMD.
I was brave and had many tests.
She gave my parents some advice,
so they could help me feel at my best.

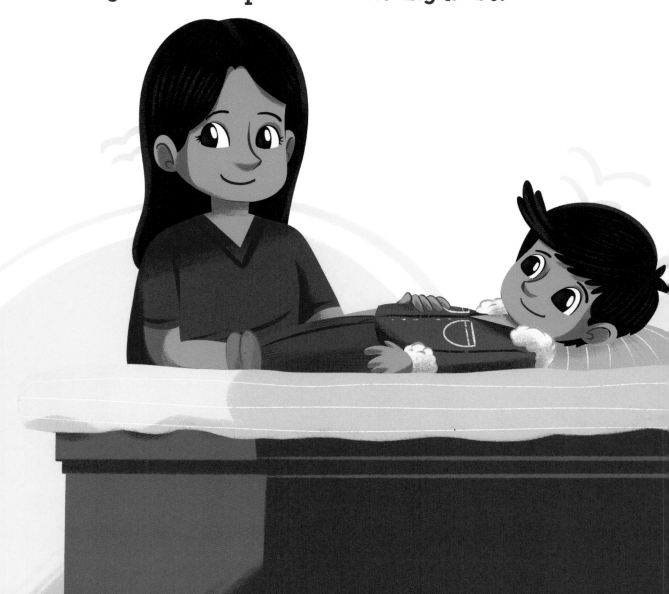

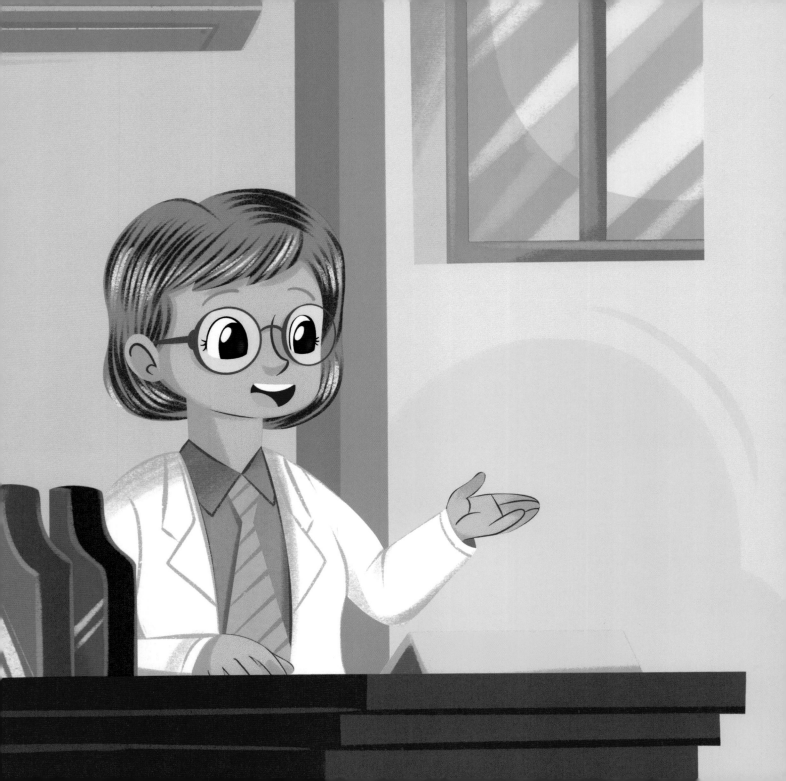

This condition is most common in children,
which can appear from the age of two.
If you have got Duchenne muscular dystrophy,
I am going through this with you!

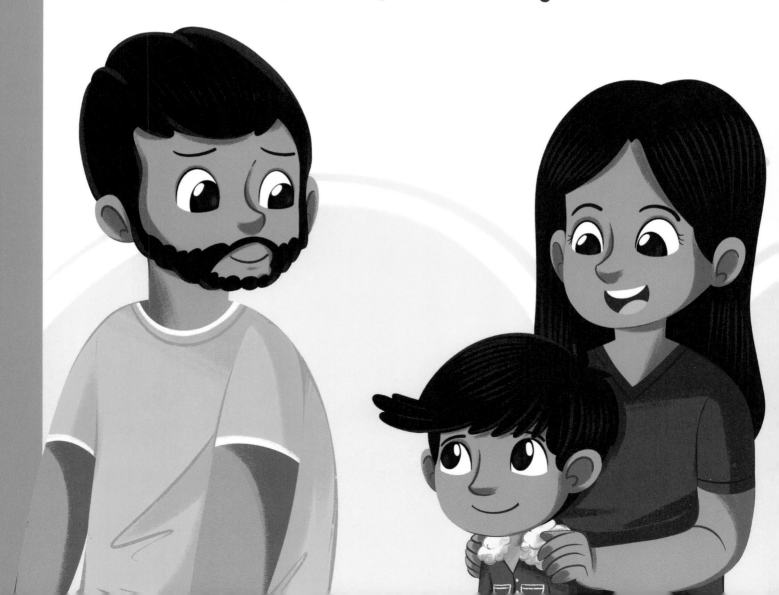

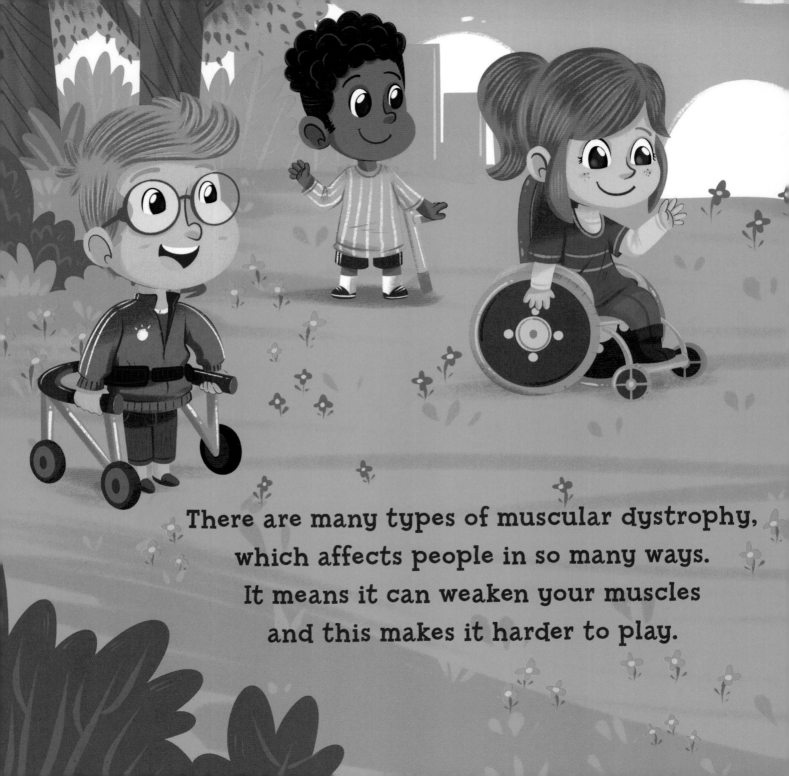

There are many types of muscular dystrophy,
which affects people in so many ways.
It means it can weaken your muscles
and this makes it harder to play.

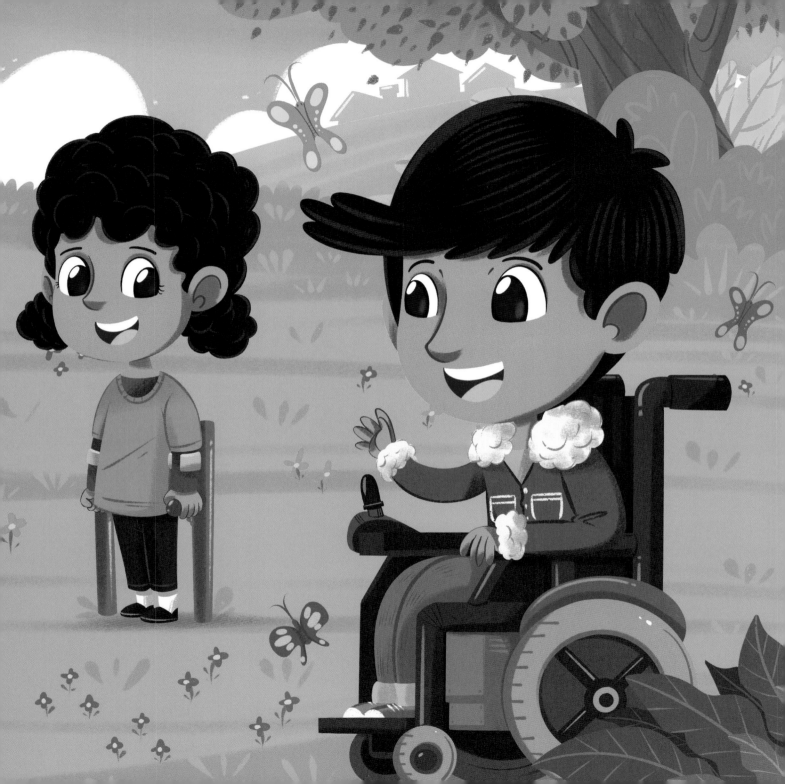

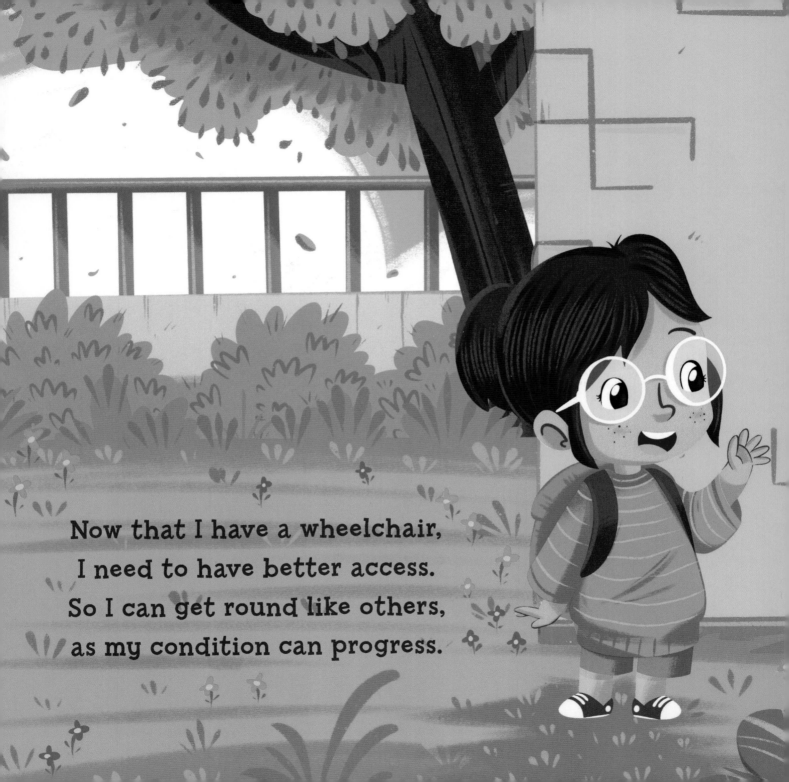

Now that I have a wheelchair,
I need to have better access.
So I can get round like others,
as my condition can progress.

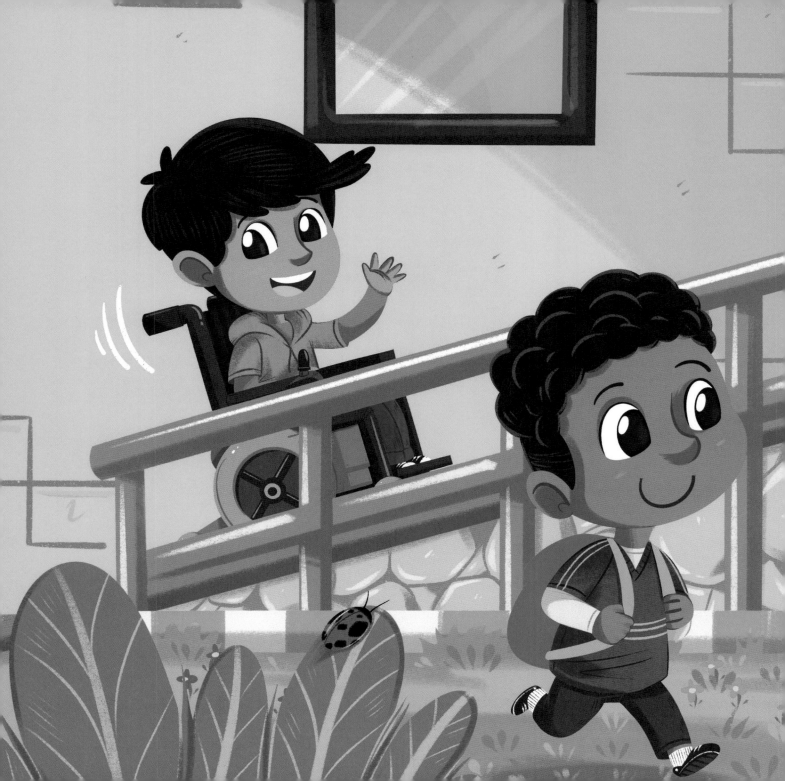

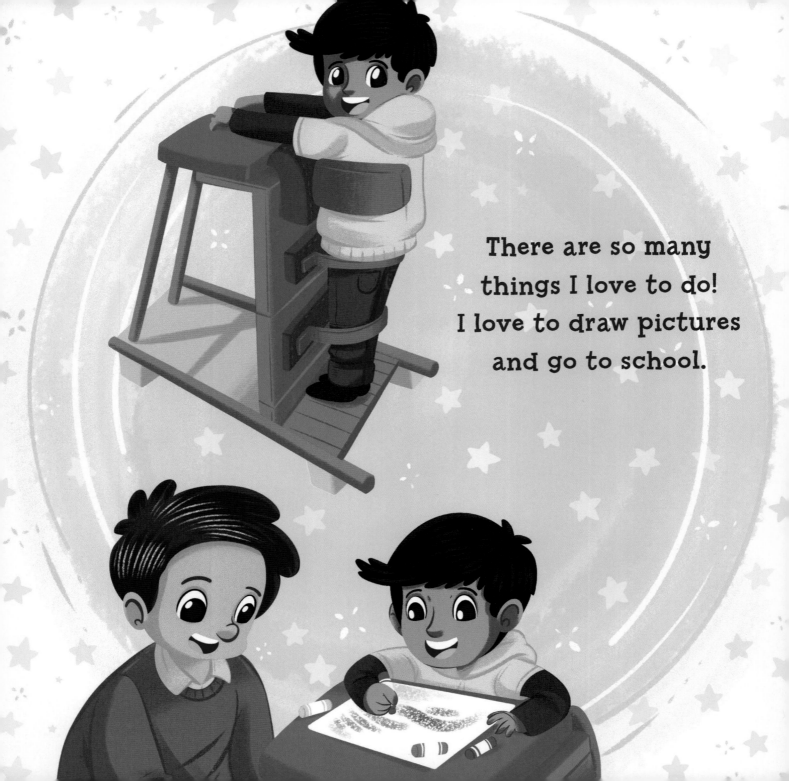

There are so many things I love to do! I love to draw pictures and go to school.

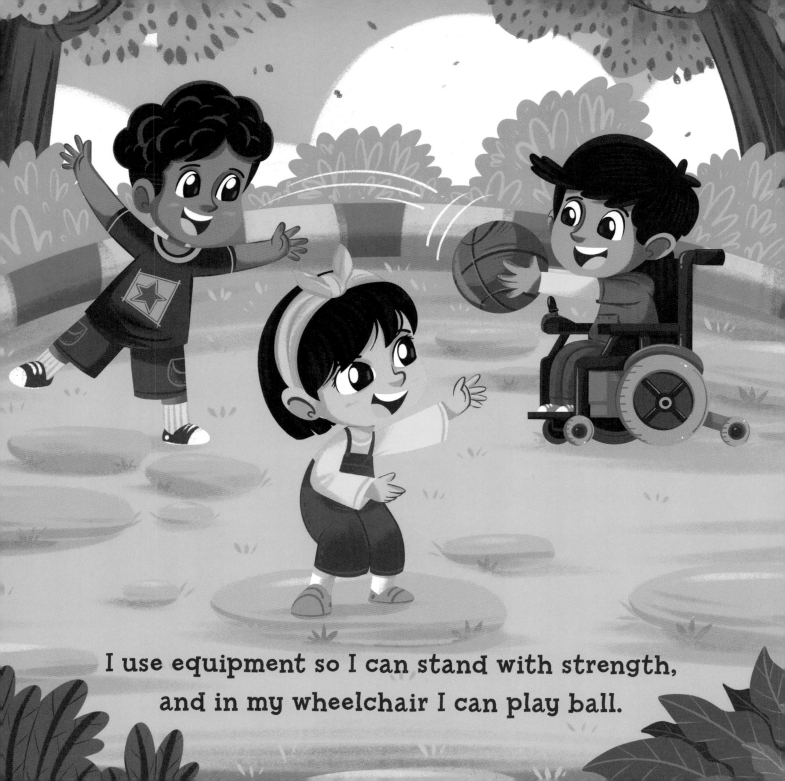

I use equipment so I can stand with strength,
and in my wheelchair I can play ball.

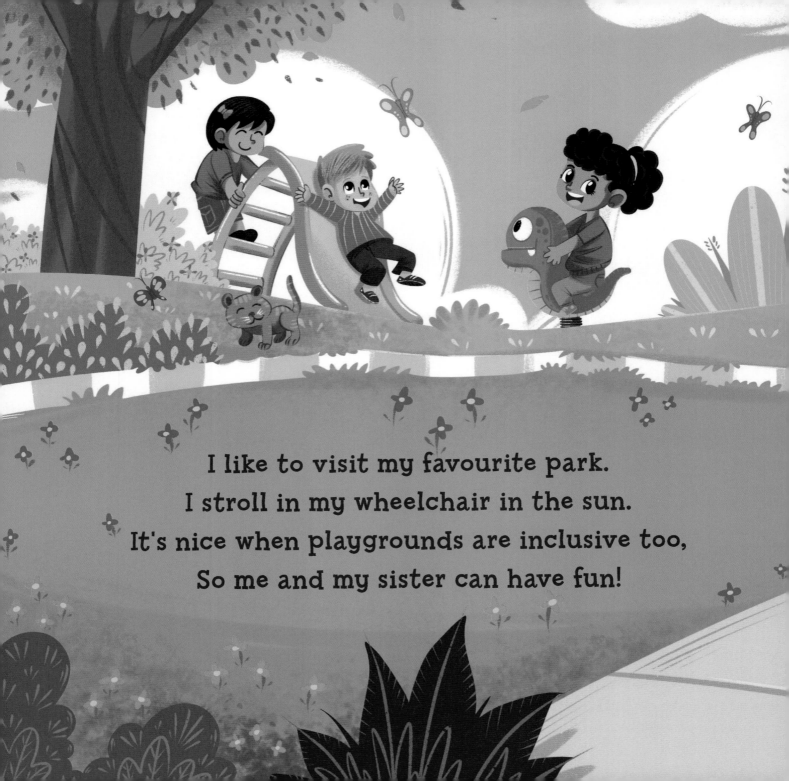

I like to visit my favourite park.
I stroll in my wheelchair in the sun.
It's nice when playgrounds are inclusive too,
So me and my sister can have fun!

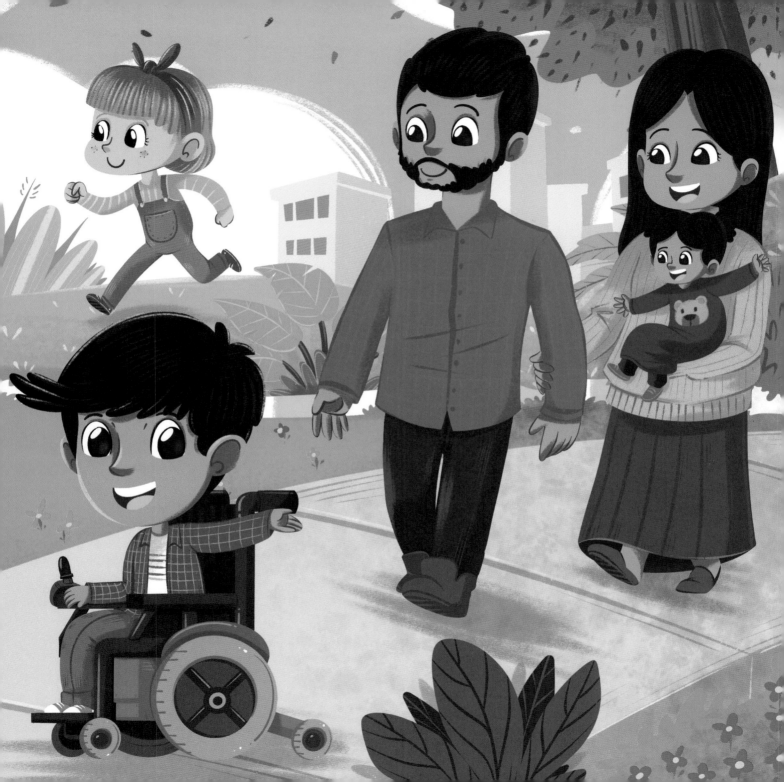

I love to spend days out with my family,
my father carries me over the sand.

My family make me feel so loved,
being together hand in hand.

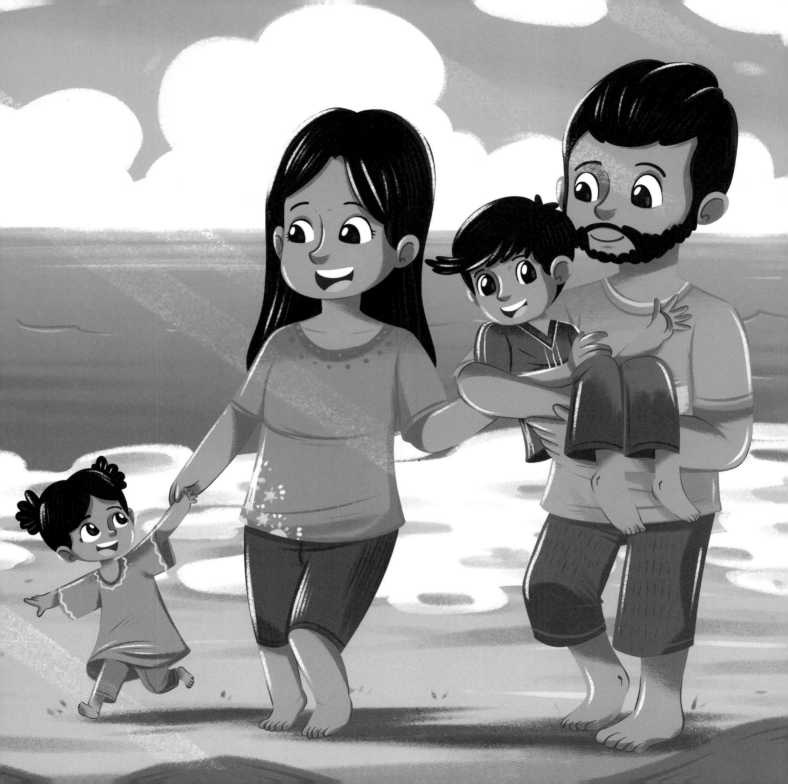

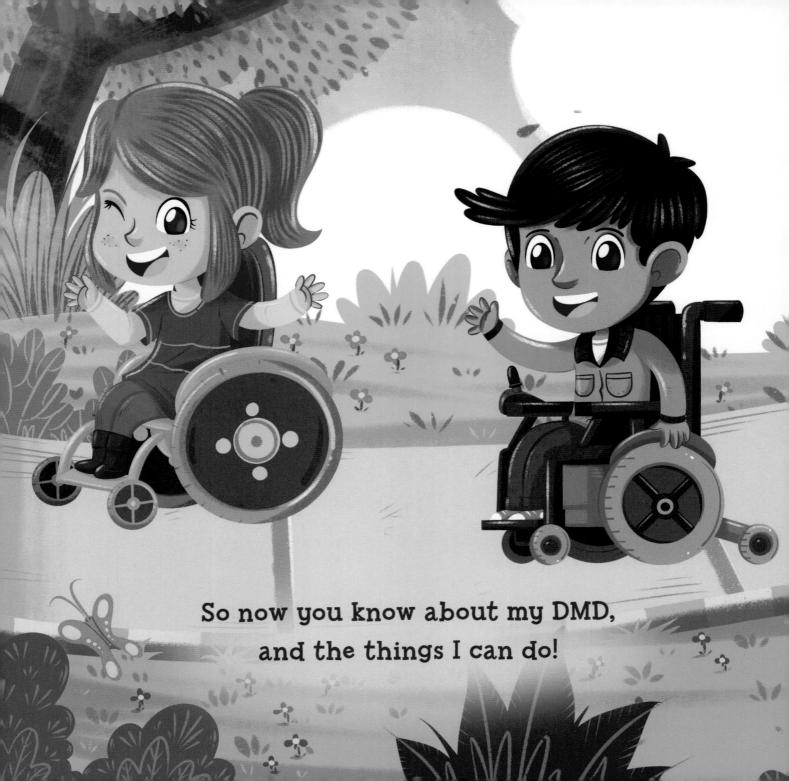

So now you know about my DMD,
and the things I can do!

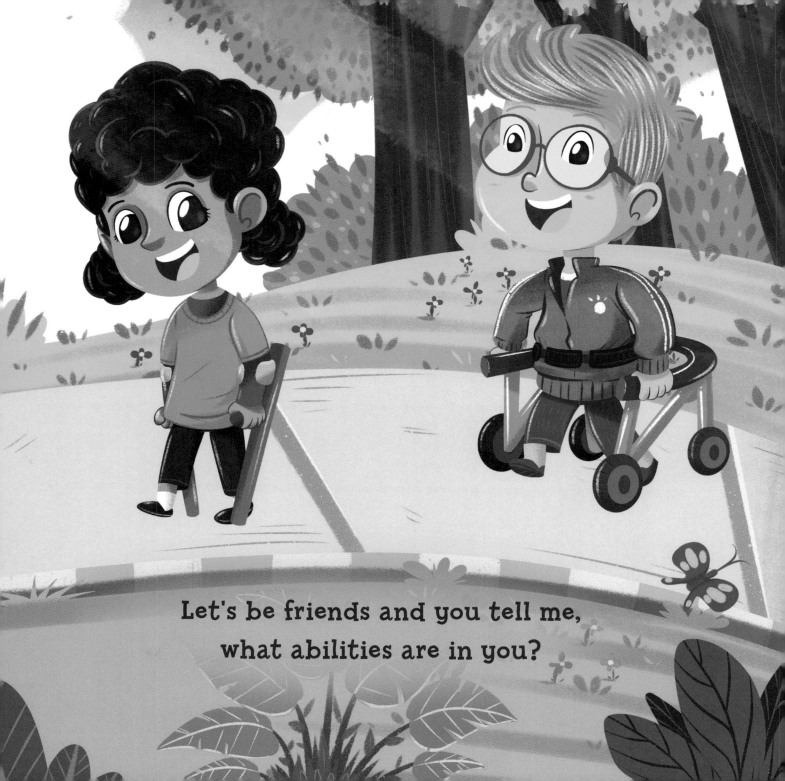

Let's be friends and you tell me,
what abilities are in you?

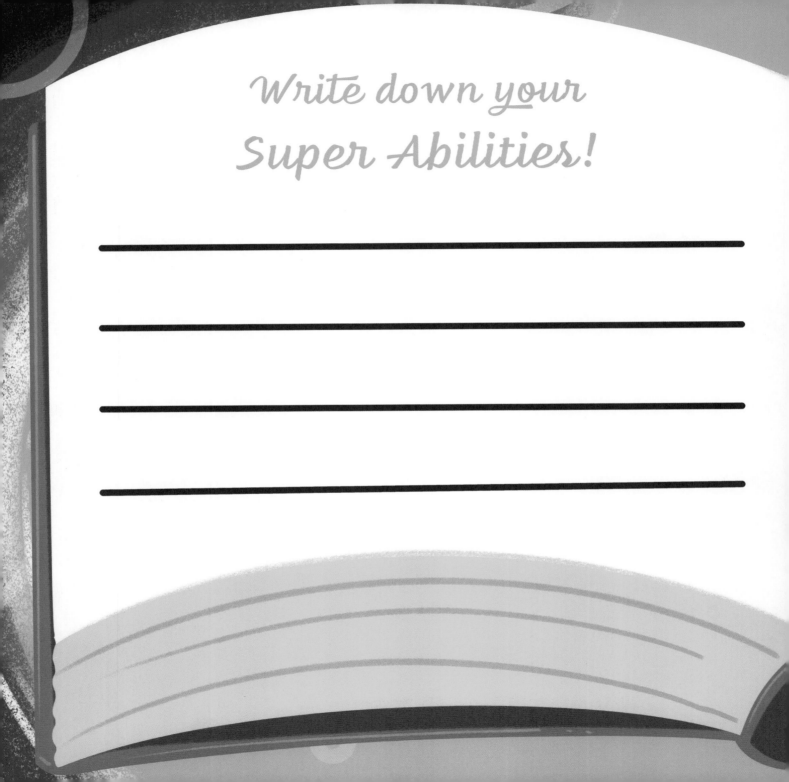

Write down your Super Abilities!

What makes you Happy?
Please draw below!

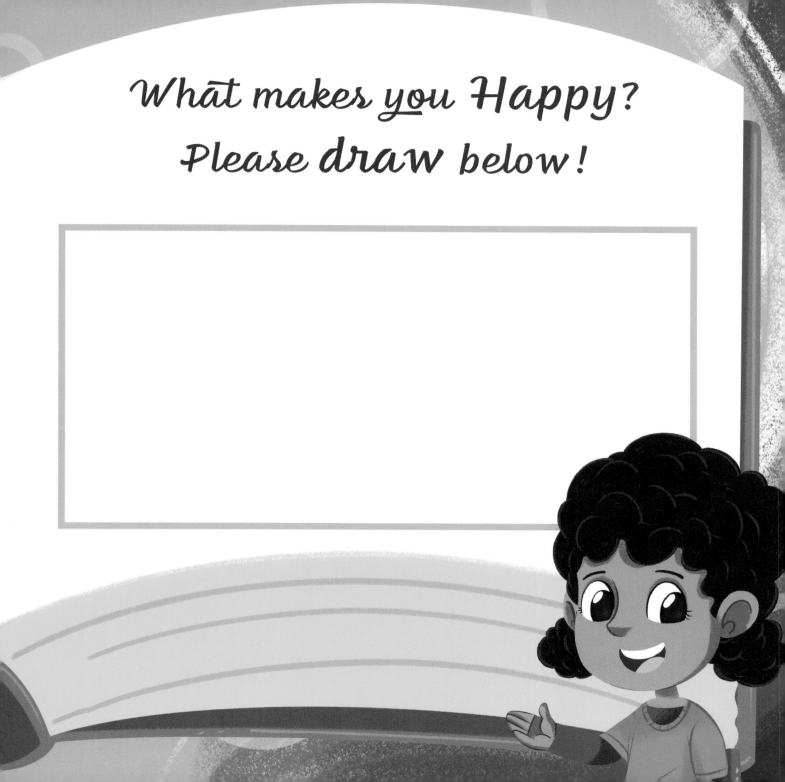

Support Information

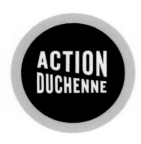

Formed in 2001, **Action Duchenne** was the first UK charity dedicated to supporting those living with Duchenne muscular dystrophy. We are a community-led charity, putting our Duchenne young people, adults and their families at the forefront to meet their needs.

We have three core objectives and are proud that 87p in every £1 raised is spent on our charitable activities:

- Funding research for everyone living with Duchenne
- Cutting-edge science education programmes
- World-class support for Duchenne families

Charity number - Registered Charity Number: 1101971 Scotland: SC043852

Website and social media links for family support:

www.actionduchenne.org

- ActionDuchenne
- ActionDuchenne
- info@actionduchenne.org

Support Information

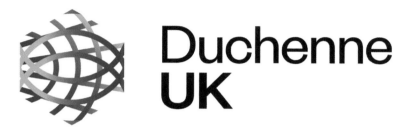

Duchenne UK is the leading charity in the UK for Duchenne muscular dystrophy research. We're going further to find effective treatments for DMD to end its devastating impact. We're doing it faster, too, by accelerating access to these treatments and therapies for this generation of patients. And we're here to support every family affected and ensure that they receive the best possible care.

www.duchenneuk.org

🅕 duchenneuk

🅞 duchenneuk

🅣 duchenneuk

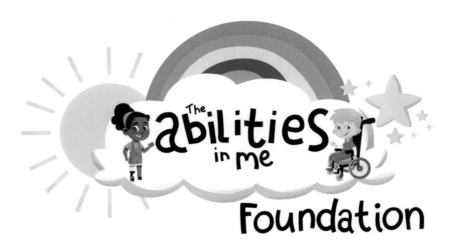

The Abilities in Me Foundation aims to raise awareness of special educational needs and conditions that children may encounter. We have an ever-growing book series written for young people that celebrates what these children can do, rather than what they cannot do. The Foundation also provides community support through forums and special events and works with schools to deliver educational workshops.

At the Abilities in Me, we want all children, regardless of their barriers to feel accepted and understood. The books are inspired by real children and experiences and they enable parents and teachers to talk about different needs and conditions with their children in a fun, safe and engaging way.

Our book series has had such a positive impact on children around the world and we will continue to widen our range and encourage further research and funding into different conditions. The Abilities in Me Foundation aims to raise funds to support worthy causes and by bringing awareness into schools, we hope that this will encourage kindness and reduce bullying.

Find out more information via our website **www.theabilitiesinme.com**
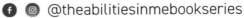 @theabilitiesinmebookseries

Check out our bookshelf!

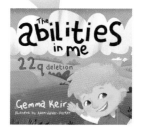 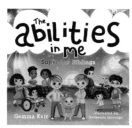 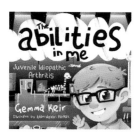 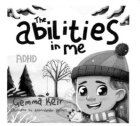 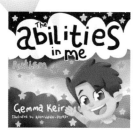

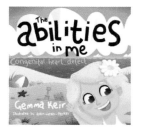 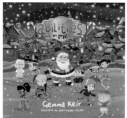 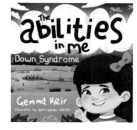 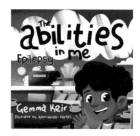 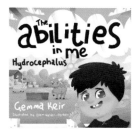

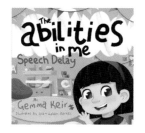 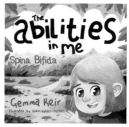 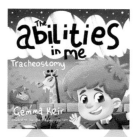 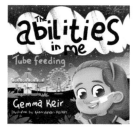 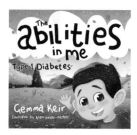

available at
amazon